# HEALING YOUR SKIN AILMENTS

A Comprehensive Guide to Living Life Comfortably And Free of Skin Issues

Dr. Vivian L. Martinez

Chapter 1: Introduction

Chapter 2: Causes of Skin Ailments
1. Poor Diet
2. Environmental Factors
3. Genetics, 4. Stress
5. Hormones

Chapter 3: Natural Remedies

1. Hydration

2. Healthy Diet

3. Sun Protection

4. Stress Management

5. Exercise

6. Herbal Remedies

Chapter 4: Medical Treatments

1. Topical Medications

2. Oral Medications

3. Light Therapy

4. Surgical Procedures

Chapter 5: Conclusion

Copyright © 2022 by [Dr. Vivian L. Martinez] All rights reserved. No part of this book may be reproduced in any form or by any electronic or mechanical means, including information storage and retrieval systems, without permission in writing from the publisher, except by a reviewer who may quote brief passages in a review.

This book is a work of nonfiction. The names, characters, places, and incidents are products of the author's imagination or are used fictitiously. Any resemblance to actual events, locales, or persons, living or dead, is coincidental.

First edition: 2022 [Dr. Vivian L. Martinez]

# Chapter 1

Introduction

Jennifer had always struggled with problematic skin. She had tried countless skincare products and treatments over the years, but nothing seemed to work. She was constantly dealing with breakouts, redness, and irritation, which was starting to take a toll on her confidence.

One day, Jennifer decided to take a different approach. She started researching natural skincare remedies and began experimenting with other ingredients. Jennifer started using honey as a face mask, applying it to her skin and leaving it on for 15 minutes before rinsing it off. She also began using tea tree oil to spot and treat any blemishes and made sure to eat and drink lots of water—a healthy diet.

Slowly but surely, Jennifer's skin started to improve. The honey helped to soothe and moisturize her skin, while the tea tree oil helped to fight bacteria and clear up any breakouts. She also noticed that her skin was less red and irritated and she felt more confident and comfortable.

As time went on, Jennifer continued to experiment with different natural skincare remedies, and she found a routine that worked for her. She finally said goodbye to her skin ailments and embraced her beautiful, healthy skin.

Welcome! This journey of healing your skin ailments starts with you. Here, you will learn how to nourish and protect your skin; choosing the ideal products for your skin type involves managing flare-ups and other skin issues. By taking the time to understand your skin's needs and arming yourself with the knowledge to support it, you will be on your way to a healthier, more beautiful complexion.

A healthy, glowing complexion is not only a sign of physical health but can also boost your confidence and self-esteem. However, many of us struggle with various skin ailments, such as acne, dryness, and discoloration, that can leave our skin damaged and unbalanced. Fortunately, there are many ways to heal and rejuvenate your skin, and it all starts with taking a holistic approach to your skincare routine.

By nourishing your body from the inside out, using natural, gentle skincare products, and making simple lifestyle changes, you can restore balance and radiance to your skin and improve its overall health and appearance. With commitment and consistency, you can say goodbye to skin ailments and hello to a beautiful, healthy complexion. So let's begin!

# Chapter 2

Causes of skin ailments

**1. Poor Diet**

It can reflect Poor nutrition in the skin. A bad diet can bring on skin conditions like dryness, peeling, wrinkles, and acne.

Skin imbalance can result from a diet lacking vital vitamins and minerals. Vitamin deficits can result in dryness and wrinkles since vitamins A, C, and E are essential for healthy skin. Deficiencies in omega-3 fatty acids, zinc, and selenium can cause rosacea, eczema, and acne. These nutrients are also necessary for good skin.

Saturated fats, sugary beverages, and processed food-heavy diets can all harm the health of your skin. These foods can aggravate skin disorders like acne, psoriasis, and dermatitis. Fresh fruits and vegetables, along with a diet low in processed foods, can help to support good skin.

Water consumption is also crucial for healthy skin. Water can help keep the skin hydrated and prevent dryness while aiding the body's detoxification process.

The condition of your skin also depends on getting adequate sleep. Dark circles, bags, and wrinkles can result from sleep deprivation.

## 2. Environmental Factors

Environmental factors that affect skin conditions include exposure to pollutants, temperature and humidity variations, and allergens such as dust mites or pollen.

Skin diseases like eczema and psoriasis can develop as a result of irritation and inflammation brought on by exposure to tobacco smoke, air pollution, and other environmental contaminants.

Changes in humidity and temperature can make skin dry and itchy, aggravate eczema and psoriasis, and raise the risk of fungal infections.

Sunburns and long-term skin damage from UV radiation can result in early aging and a higher chance of developing skin cancer.

Contact dermatitis, an itchy rash brought on by an allergen, can be brought on by allergens such as dust mites, pollen, and animal dander.

Skin irritation and sensitivity can also be brought on by exposure to specific chemicals, such as those included in cosmetics and cleaning goods.

Finally, stress can cause skin problems, including acne, psoriasis, and hives.

People can lower their chance of acquiring skin disorders by adopting measures to decrease exposure to environmental variables, such as reducing exposure to air pollution, using sunscreen, and avoiding allergies.

## 3. Genetics

Dermatogenetics, another name for the area of medicine that prioritizes the study of the genetic elements that influence the development of skin problems, is the genetics of skin conditions. Many skin disorders, including eczema, acne, and psoriasis, have a genetic component that makes certain people more prone to developing these conditions.

The generation of aberrant proteins or enzymes that impact the skin's composition and functionality is one way that hereditary factors might contribute to the emergence of skin diseases. For instance, changes in the gene that makes the filaggrin enzyme may impair the protein's capacity to maintain the skin's barrier function, resulting in diseases like eczema.

Through the immune system, heredity can also influence skin conditions. Inflammation and the emergence of skin diseases like psoriasis might result from the immune system overreacting to specific triggers due to individual genetic differences.

How a person responds to skin disease treatments might also be influenced by heredity. For instance, whereas some people may have a genetic predisposition to react badly to specific treatments, others may have a genetic profile that increases their likelihood of responding favorably to therapy.

In general, the genetics of skin disorders is a challenging and developing research topic. Researchers are attempting to understand better the genetic elements that contribute to their onset to acquire more effective treatments for skin problems.

## 4. Stress

Stress is a widespread issue affecting people of all ages and socioeconomic backgrounds. It happens when a person feels that the expectations placed on them are more than their capacity to handle them. Stress can affect the body in various ways, causing physical and psychological symptoms such as irritation and difficulty concentrating. Physical symptoms include headaches and stomachaches.

Skill illnesses are one of the most typical ways that stress shows itself. These are difficulties carrying out duties or engaging in pursuits that one used to find enjoyable and straightforward. For instance, a person experiencing stress may find it challenging to focus or use their fine motor skills for activities like typing or playing an instrument.

There are numerous approaches to managing stress and avoiding skill maladies. Some people discover that stress management strategies like meditation, yoga, or counseling can help them. Others might require alterations to their way of life or place of employment to lessen the sources of stress in their lives.

It's crucial to remember that because everyone reacts to stress differently, One person's solution might not be suitable for another. Reduce your tension and avoid skill problems; the key is to develop a coping strategy that works for you and practice it frequently.

## 5. Hormones

Hormones are essential for controlling various bodily processes, including skin health. Numerous hormones can impact the skin, and hormonal imbalances can result in several skin diseases.

Estrogen is one of the hormones that is known to have an impact on the skin. The ovaries create the female sex hormone known as estrogen. It controls several facets of female physiology, including the skin's condition. During menopause, estrogen levels often decrease, which can cause dry, thin skin and an increase in wrinkles. The use of estrogen replacement treatment can assist in balancing hormones and enhance skin health.

Androgen is a different hormone that has an impact on the skin. The hormone responsible for the male sex, androgen, is created by the testes. The ovaries and the adrenal glands both produce androgen in females. Sebum is an oily material that aids in maintaining the moisture of the skin, and androgen plays a part in controlling how much is produced. Acne may occur due to increased sebum production from an excess of androgen.

Another class of hormones that impact the skin is thyroid hormones. The thyroid gland, found in the neck, creates hormones that control how quickly the body burns through food. Thinner skin can result from an overactive thyroid gland (hyperthyroidism), and dry, rough skin might result from an underactive thyroid gland (hypothyroidism).

Overall, hormones are essential in controlling skin health. Hormone imbalances can cause various skin disorders, and correcting these imbalances can help the skin stay healthy.

# Chapter 3

**Natural Remedies**

**1. Hydration**

The process of hydrating involves supplying moisture to the skin. It is an essential component of skin care since the skin needs adequate hydration to keep its elasticity, suppleness, and general health.

Dehydration can cause the skin to become dry, flaky, irritable, and susceptible to various skin conditions. Eczema, psoriasis, and dermatitis are common skin problems that can be exacerbated or caused by dehydration.

Use items that help add moisture to the skin and lock it in if you want to hydrate your skin properly. It can include serums, moisturizers, and other skin care items created to hydrate the skin.

The general health and hydration of the skin can be supported by drinking lots of water and eating a nutritious diet high in fruits and vegetables. Using delicate items that prevent removing the skin's natural oils and avoiding abrasive soaps and cleansers can also assist in keeping the skin adequately hydrated.

In conclusion, proper hydration is crucial for maintaining healthy, elastic skin free from common skin conditions. You can assist in keeping your skin properly hydrated and looking its best by using the right products, consuming enough water, and adhering to a healthy skincare routine.

## 2. Healthy Diet

Eating a balanced diet is crucial for maintaining general health and well-being and can help treat skin issues. Certain foods, such as those high in vitamins, minerals, and other nutrients that support healthy skin, are particularly good for the skin.

Vitamin A, which foods such as sweet potatoes and carrots include spinach, and kale, is one of the most crucial vitamins for good skin. Vitamin A can keep the skin healthy and looking smooth and supple by preserving its integrity. Vitamin C is vital for healthy skin to increase collagen production and shield the skin from free radical damage. Oranges, strawberries, and bell peppers are a few foods high in vitamin C.

Several minerals are also crucial for good skin, in addition to vitamins. For instance, zinc can aid in reducing skin inflammation and speeding up wound healing. Oysters, steak, and chicken are among the foods high in zinc. Another essential mineral for good skin is selenium, which can help shield the skin from ultraviolet (UV) light damage. Selenium-rich foods include Brazil nuts, tuna, and chicken.

Omega-3 fatty acids are another essential ingredient for good skin; they can aid in lowering inflammation and encourage healthy skin cell proliferation. Omega-3 fatty acids are found in foods like flaxseeds, chia seeds, walnuts, and rich seafood like salmon, mackerel, and herring.

Lean proteins, whole grains, and a range of fruits and vegetables should all be part of a nutritious diet to maintain healthy skin. Additionally, it's critical to avoid processed meals and sugary beverages, which can exacerbate inflammation and other skin issues, and to consume lots of water to keep the skin hydrated. You can keep your skin healthy and bright by consuming a balanced diet and taking care of it.

## 3. Sun Protection

Sun protection ought to be a top concern for anyone who wishes to keep their skin in good condition. Sun damage is one of the leading causes of skin conditions like early aging, wrinkles, sunburns, and skin cancer. Use sunscreen daily, dress in protective gear, and Avoid being in the sun for as long as possible.

Your skin needs sunscreen to be shielded from the damaging UV rays of the sun radiation. All exposed skin should have sunscreen applied liberally and uniformly and used again after swimming, sweating, towel drying, or every two hours. Make careful to choose a broad-spectrum sunblock with a minimum SPF of 30.

Wearing protective clothing can help lower your risk of UV damage in addition to using sunscreen. A light, loose-fitting outfit that covers most of your skin is preferred. Sunglasses and a wide-brimmed hat can both help to further reduce sun exposure.

Finally, limiting how much time is spent outdoors in the sun is essential, especially in the middle of the day. When feasible, seek shade and stay indoors between 10 am and 4 pm.

**4. Stress Management**

Your skin's health can be significantly impacted by stress. When under pressure, your body creates hormones like cortisol, which can exacerbate inflammatory skin diseases like acne, eczema, and psoriasis. Maintaining your physical and mental wellness is crucial for managing stress and enhancing the quality of your skin. Here are some pointers for reducing stress and improving skin health:

- Practice relaxation methods: Try incorporating relaxation methods into your routines, such as deep breathing exercises, meditation, or yoga. These pursuits can assist in calming the mind and lowering the release of stress hormones.

- Sleep well: Sleep is essential for maintaining healthy skin. Your body can repair and replace skin cells better when you get enough sleep. Sleep for 7-9 hours every night. for good skin.

- Maintain a healthy diet: Eating many processed and sugary foods can worsen skin issues and cause inflammation. Focus on eating a balanced diet high in fruits, vegetables, and healthy fats.

- To keep your skin hydrated and healthy, drink a lot of water throughout the day. Drinking water may keep your skin looking young and radiant and aid in the removal of toxins.

- Avoid harsh skincare products because they can dry up and irritate your skin, making it more prone to flare-ups brought on by stress. Choose gentle, all-natural cosmetics that will nourish and protect your skin instead.

You may contribute to the improvement of the health of your skin and lessen the adverse effects of stress on your body by adopting these stress management practices into your daily routine.

## 5. Exercise

An excellent way to enhance the health of your skin is through exercise. Your body boosts blood flow to your skin when you exercise, which may aid in hydrating and oxygenating your skin cells. Your skin's overall health and look can both be enhanced by doing this.

Exercise can also aid in lowering stress, a common cause of many skin conditions like eczema and acne. You can lessen the frequency and severity of certain skin disorders by exercising to reduce stress.

Stretching, strength training, and aerobics are some exercise styles that might be good for your skin. Finding an exercise program that you like and that fits into your lifestyle is crucial if you want to stick with it and see positive results for your skin.

In addition to exercising, it's critical to take good care of your skin by using healthy skincare practices. Regular skin cleansing, mild, non-irritating treatments, and sun protection are all part of this. Regular exercise and proper skincare practices can work together to keep your skin looking and feeling its best.

## 6. Herbal Remedies

Numerous skin conditions have been treated with herbal treatments for ages. Numerous plants have natural anti-inflammatory and therapeutic characteristics that can aid in calming sensitive skin and hasten the healing process. Chamomile, aloe vera, and calendula are a few herbs frequently used to treat skin conditions.

A well-liked herb with relaxing and anti-inflammatory qualities is chamomile.

Eczema, psoriasis, and other skin disorders that produce redness and irritation are frequently treated with it. Make chamomile tea by steeping the herb in hot water, then use a cotton ball to apply the cooled tea to the afflicted area as a natural skin cure. You can also buy chamomile oil or ointment at your neighborhood health food store and apply it to the skin.

Another herb that is frequently used to treat skin issues is aloe vera. Aloe vera plant gel has a cooling impact on the skin and can assist in easing sunburns and minimizing swelling. Additionally, you can use it to treat scrapes, cuts, and other minor skin wounds. Break off a portion of the plant and squeeze the gel onto the injured area to utilize aloe vera as a natural skin cure.

Herbs like calendula usually referred to as pot marigold, are frequently utilized in organic skin care products. Acne, eczema, and rashes can all be effectively treated with it since it has anti-inflammatory and antibacterial characteristics. You can apply Calendula oil or ointment directly to the affected area, or the herb can be steeped in hot water to form a tea that can be used on the skin once it has cooled.

In conclusion, using herbal treatments to treat various skin conditions can be prosperous and healthy. Some of the most popular herbs for skin care include chamomile, aloe vera, and calendula, which can relieve irritation, lessen inflammation, and hasten the healing process. Always get medical advice before using herbal treatments, especially if you are expecting or already have a medical condition.

# Chapter 4

**Medical Treatment**

1. Topical Medication

Direct application of topical medicines to the skin and treat various skin conditions. These medications can be used in creams, gels, ointments, or lotions and can treat everything from mild skin irritation to more severe conditions like acne and eczema.

One of the most common topical medications used to treat skin conditions is corticosteroids. These drugs are anti-inflammatory and can help to reduce swelling, redness, and itching. They are often used to treat conditions like eczema, dermatitis, and psoriasis.

Another type of topical medication commonly used to treat skin conditions is retinoids. These drugs are derived from vitamin A and can help unclog pores, reduce inflammation, and improve the skin's overall appearance. They are often used to treat conditions like acne and can also lessen the visibility of wrinkles and fine lines.

Topical antibiotics are also commonly used to treat certain skin conditions. These drugs are applied directly to the skin and can help to kill bacteria that can cause infections and inflammation. They are often used to treat conditions like acne and can be combined with other medications for greater effectiveness.

Overall, topical medications can be a successful method to treat a variety of range of skin conditions. They are typically applied to the affected area and can relieve symptoms like swelling, redness, and itching. It is essential to follow the medication label instructions and consult with a medical professional if you have any queries or worries.

## 2. Oral Medication

Oral medications are taken by mouth instead of applied directly to the skin. These medications often treat skin diseases such as psoriasis, eczema, and acne.
One common oral medication used to treat acne is isotretinoin, a form of vitamin A. Isotretinoin helps reduce sebum production. This natural oil can clog pores and lead to acne. It also helps to reduce the growth of bacteria on the skin, which can cause acne.

Another common oral medication used to treat eczema and psoriasis is a class of drugs known as corticosteroids. These drugs reduce inflammation in the skin, which can help relieve the redness, itching, and swelling associated with these conditions.
It's important to note that you should only take oral medications for skin conditions under the guidance of a healthcare provider.

These medications can have side effects, and monitoring for potential adverse reactions is essential. Sometimes, a combination of oral and topical medications may be necessary to treat a skin condition effectively.

## 3. Light Therapy

A treatment option is a light therapy, also referred to as phototherapy, which uses different wavelengths of light to treat various skin conditions. It is a standard treatment option for conditions such as acne, eczema, and psoriasis.
During light therapy, the patient stands or sits in front of a light. Therapy box that emits either natural sunlight or artificial light. The light is absorbed by the skin and can help to kill bacteria, reduce inflammation, and improve overall skin health.
Light therapy is typically safe and well-tolerated, although Some persons could have adverse effects like redness, itching, or

dryness. It is essential to follow the rules. A healthcare provider, when using a light therapy box, overexposure to light can cause damage to the skin.

In addition to treating skin conditions, light therapy has also been shown to treat certain forms of depression and seasonal affective disorder (SAD). You can use it alone or with other treatments, such as medication or talk therapy.

Light therapy is a safe and effective treatment option for various skin conditions and can help improve overall skin health and appearance.

**4. Surgical Procedures**

Can use Various surgical procedures to treat skin ailments. Some common ones include:

- Excision: This is an operation where the doctor removes the entire skin lesion (such as a mole or skin growth) and a margin of healthy skin around it. The doctor then closes the wound with stitches or staples.

- Incision and drainage: This is a surgical procedure used to treat abscesses (collections of pus) or cysts (tiny, fluid-filled sacs) in the skin. The physician creates a slight wound in the skin and drains the pus or fluid from the abscess or cyst. The damage is then cleaned and covered with a dressing.

- Mohs surgery is a specialized surgical procedure for handling skin malignancies like squamous and basal cells.65 The doctor removes the cancerous tissue layer by layer, using a microscope to check each layer for cancer cells. It allows the doctor to remove as little healthy tissue as possible while ensuring that all cancerous tissue is removed.

- Grafts and flaps: These are surgical procedures in which healthy skin is transferred from one bodily component to another.

Grafts involve removing a piece of healthy skin and attaching it to the wound, while flaps involve moving a bit of skin along with the blood vessels that supply it with blood. Using grafts and flaps, one can have large wounds or areas of missing skin.

Overall, the type of surgical procedure used to treat a skin ailment will depend on the specific condition and the doctor's preference. It's essential to consult with a qualified healthcare professional to determine the best treatment option for your situation.

# Chapter 5

**Conclusion**

Skin ailments can cause significant discomfort and distress for those suffering from them. It is essential to seek medical advice and follow a treatment plan if you experience any symptoms associated with a skin ailment. While there is no guaranteed cure, many skin ailments can be managed with proper diagnosis and treatment, allowing those affected to live their lives with minimal disruption and discomfort.

Skin ailments can be concerning and even debilitating. However, skin ailments can be managed and eliminated with the right treatment plan, lifestyle changes, and skincare routine. If you are experiencing any skin issues, it's essential to seek medical advice to ensure that your skin gets the proper care it needs. With the right help, you can relieve skin ailments and restore your skin's health.

In conclusion, skin ailments can range from minor ailments that are simple to treat to serious ones. and chronic diseases. It is essential to regularly monitor and care for the skin to prevent and treat these conditions. Seeking medical advice from a dermatologist can help diagnose and manage skin ailments effectively. Proper skincare and healthy lifestyle habits can also help prevent the development of skin ailments.

www.ingramcontent.com/pod-product-compliance
Lightning Source LLC
Chambersburg PA
CBHW050323220526
45465CB00005B/2102